I0695722

TABLE OF CONTENTS

INTRODUCTION

Many parents easily recognize the physical needs of their child when it comes to providing adequate healthy food, water, and a secure environment. But once it comes to the mental health of the child, parents find it difficult to recognize it. A child's mental health may not be as noticeable as his or her physical condition or needs; as a result, before even attempting to understand the child's progress, the parent must be conversant on the subject of mental health development and cultural diversity.

Culture directly influences how we see particular ideas or behaviors, and it can have many negative or positive effects on our mental health. It can affect many things, including how we may decide to seek treatment for mental health issues, as well as other things.

This information is not presented by a medical expert and is only for educational and informational purposes. The content is not proposed to be a substitute for professional medical advice, diagnosis or treatment. Please seek the advice of your physician or other experienced health service providers with any question you may have regarding any medical condition. Never ignore professional medical advice or hesitate in seeking it because of something you have read.

CHAPTER ONE

WHAT IS MENTAL HEALTH?

Mental health comprises emotional, psychological, and social well-being, influencing cognition, behavior and perception. It likewise decides how an individual handles stress, decision-making and interpersonal relationships. Mental health includes subjective well-being, perceived self-efficacy, intergenerational dependence, competence, autonomy and self-actualization of one's intellectual and emotional potential, among others.

World Health Organization (WHO) defines health as:

.....a state of complete physical, mental and social well-being and not merely the absence of disease or infirmity (WHO 2001, p.1).

This definition shows three ideas fundamental to the enhancement of health: mental health is an integral part of health, mental health is more than the absence of illness, and mental health is connected with physical health and behavior.

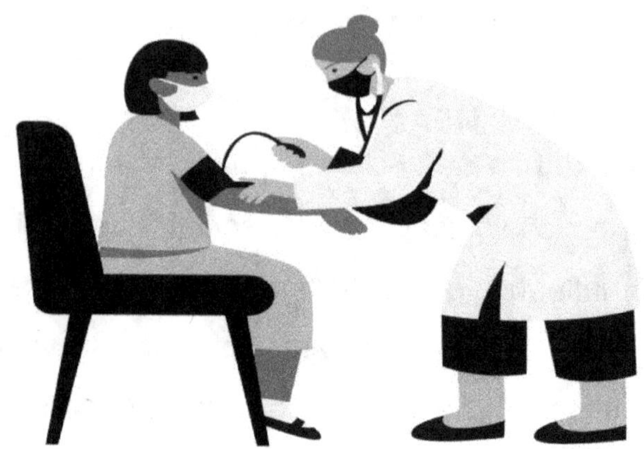

From the perspective of positive psychology, mental health may include an individual's ability to enjoy life and maintain a balance between life activities and efforts to achieve psychological flexibility.

Cultural diversity, personal assessments, and competing professional theories all affect how one defines "mental health.

Some early signs related to mental health complications are lack of energy, appetite, sleep irritation and thinking of hurting yourself or others.

CHILDREN'S MENTAL HEALTH BASICS

An ideal good mental health condition is when the child is able to think clearly in social settings and learn new skills to adapt to the needs of the surrounding at that particular time, to be able to develop his or her own self-confidence comfortably, high self-esteem and an emotionally healthy outlook on life.

WHAT IS CHILDREN'S MENTAL HEALTH?

Reaching developmental and emotional milestones, acquiring positive common skills, and learning how to cope with challenges are all part of growing up mental wellness.

Children who are mentally healthy enjoy life more and are better able to succeed at home, at school, and in every sphere of life.

Severe deviations from how kids generally learn, act, or manage their emotions are referred to as mental disorders in children. These deviations give rise to suffering and make daily life more difficult for the child.

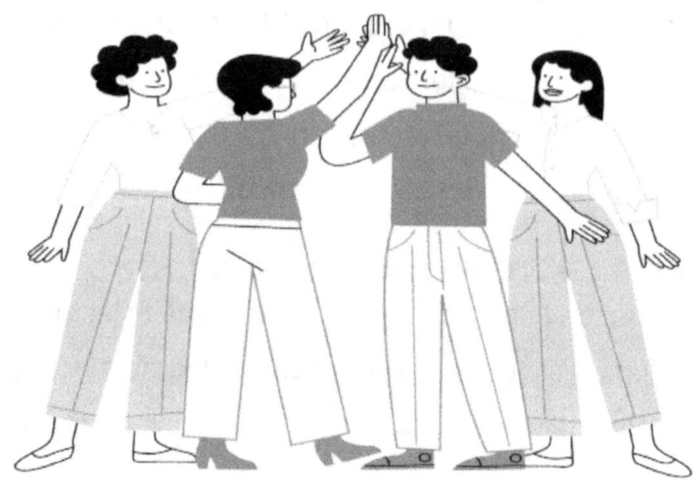

Many children frequently experience worries and fears or display unusual behaviors. If symptoms are severe and persistent and interfere with their school, home, or play activities, the child may be diagnosed with a mental disorder.

Mental health is not just simply the absence of a mental disorder. A child who does not have any mental disorder might differ in how well he is doing, and a child who is diagnosed of mental illness may differ in strength and weakness on how he is developing and coping and in quality of life.

THE BASICS

Parents should be able to provide basic fundamentals for the children, that is, unconditional love, impart self-confidence and high self-esteem, encourage social interaction by spending reasonable time with them and growth so that the child will feel comfortable knowing how to extend the same to other new additions whenever and wherever introduced, as part of their quest to understand and effectively provide for the child's optimal mental development.

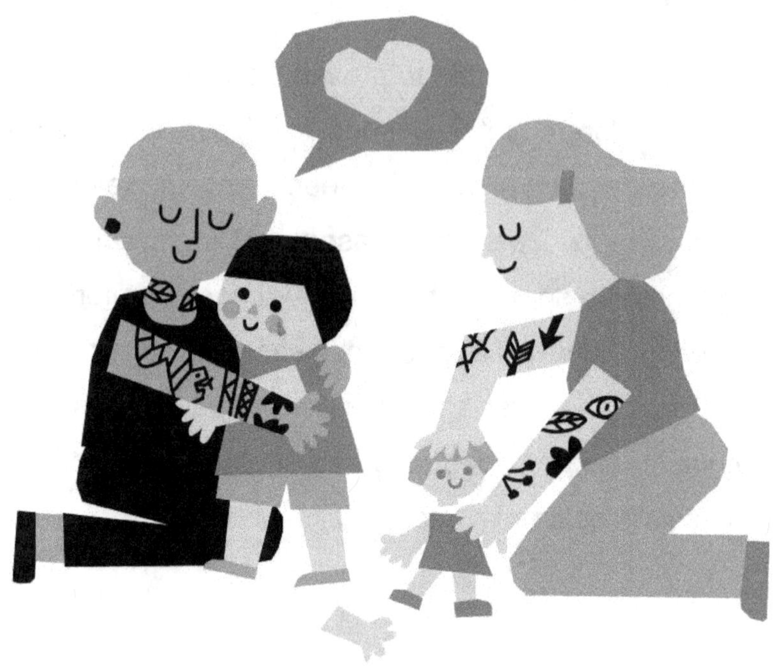

Taking reasonable time to interact with the child through play and other means of interaction, the parent will also be able to encourage the child to learn how to accept guidance and encouragement from others especially from their teachers and caregivers. This will also help the child to recognize a safe and secure environment in which to interact with others. With the appropriate guidance and discipline, the child will be able to make all the various choices required for ideal mental health growth.

CHAPTER TWO

WHY IS CHILDREN'S MENTAL HEALTH IMPORTANT?

Mental health is an important part of children's overall health and has a complex interactive relationship with their physical health and their ability to succeed in their academy, at work, and in society. Physical and mental health affect how children think, feel, and act on the inside and outside. Mental health is essential throughout childhood; from prenatal considerations through transitions to adulthood.

For instance, an overweight young boy who is teased about his weight may withdraw socially and become depressed and he may reluctant to play with or exercise with others, which may further contributes to his poorer physical health and as a result of his poorer mental health. This issue has long-term implications for the ability of children to fulfill their potential as well as consequences for the health, education, labor, and criminal justice systems of our society.

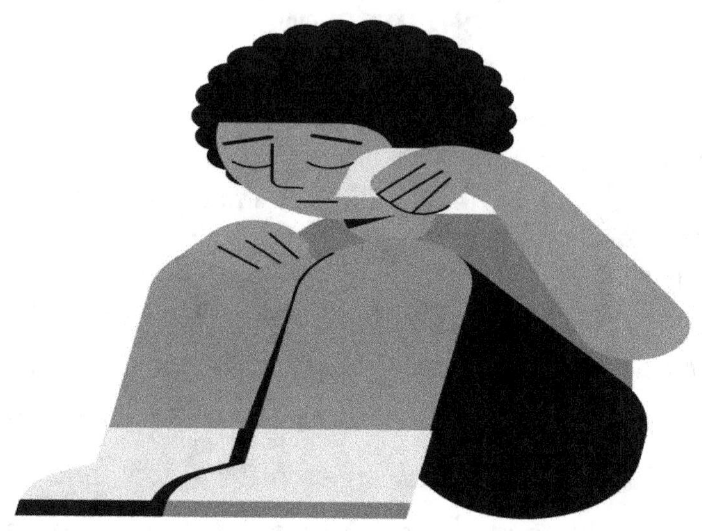

For instance, a boy who is being physically abused by his parents would often act out aggressively at school or when he is with his peer group. His behavior is a natural reaction to the abuse he received from his parents, but his behavior may also mark the beginning of an undiagnosed conduct disorder.

His teachers would simply see him as a mischief-maker and continually punish him for his behavior. Later, such child may drop out of school as a teenager because he finds it a harsh and unwelcoming environment and would be anxious to leave his abusive home and fend for himself. However, holding down a job may be difficult for such a boy because he is likely to clash with everyone at work including his supervisor or boss due to his aggression, the later end of such a boy may result in abusing alcohol and drugs which would eventually land him in the police net.

All children have the right to happy and healthy lives and deserve access to effective care to avert or treat any mental health problems that they may develop at any point in time. However, there are numerous unmet needs and health discrepancies that are particularly noticeable for children living in low-income communities, minor ethnic children, and oppressed populations such as those defined by gender identity and sexual orientation; immigration status; physical, developmental, and intellectual disabilities; or protracted medical conditions.

How Many Children Have Mental Health Disorders?

10% of children and adolescents, according to the World Health Organization (WHO), suffer from a mental disease, although the majority of them do not ask for or receive care. Lack of care toward children's and teenagers' mental health and psychosocial development has long-term effects that limit opportunities for adults to have fulfilling lives.

Globally, one in seven 10-19 years olds experiences a mental disorder, accounting for 13% of the global burden of disease in this age group.

Depression, anxiety and behavioral disorders are among the leading causes of illness and disability among adolescents.

Suicide is the fourth leading cause of death among 15-29 years-old.

Many children are at risk of developing a disorder due to risk factors in their biology or genetics; within their families, schools, and communities; and among their peers. There is a great need for mental health professionals to provide the best available culturally appropriate care based on scientific evidence, good clinical expertise, and the unique characteristics of the child. However, according to the Centers for Disease Control and Prevention, it is estimated that only about 20% of children who need services receive appropriate help from mental health professionals

What Are The Symptoms Of Childhood Mental Disorders?

Symptoms of mental disorders are not constant; they might change over time as the child grows, and may include difficulties with how the child plays, learns, speaks, and acts, or how the child handles emotions.

Symptoms often start in an early stage of childhood, although some disorders may develop during the teenage stage. The diagnosis is often made in the school years and sometimes earlier; however, some children with a mental disorder may not be recognized or diagnosed as having any.

Some of the most common mental disorders that can be diagnosed in the early childhood stage are attention-deficit/hyperactivity disorder (ADHD), anxiety (fears or worries), and behavior disorders.

Further childhood disorders and concerns that affect how children learn, behave, or handle their emotions can include learning and developmental difficulties, autism, and risk factors like substance use and self-harm.

These defects usually include cases of spina bifida, cleft palate, clubfoot and congenital dislocated hip and many other possibilities.

The defects caused by congenital infections can usually result in abnormalities when the mother experiences an infection before or during the pregnancy stage.

These infections will cause birth defects and could be in the form of rubella, cytomegalovirus, syphilis, toxoplasmosis, Venezuelan equine encephalic, parvovirus and chicken pox.

The pregnancy period is usually a stage where precautions should be taken to limit the chances of the mother having to deal with the attack of deceases that might harm the fetus.

Unfortunately, this presence of deformity is not always due to some infection as even apparently healthy parents, are occasionally presented with a child with seeming deformities.

CHAPTER THREE

Mental Health Determinants

Determinants of mental health are those factors that can enhance or pose danger to an individual's health status.

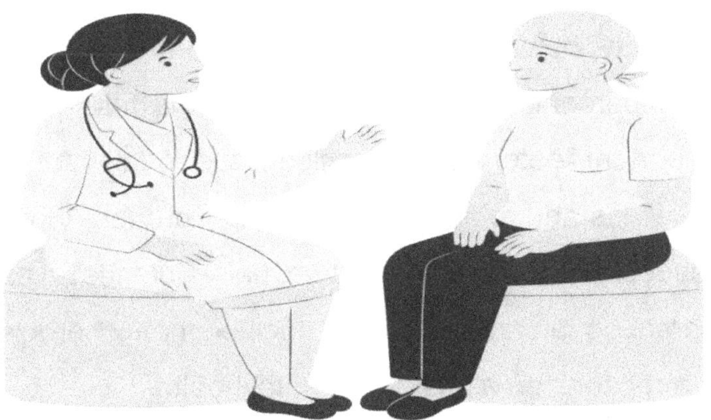

The adolescence stage is a critical time for forming social and emotional habits that are necessary for mental health. Developing, coping, problem-solving, interpersonal skills, appropriate sleep and exercise routines, and learning to control your emotions are all integral parts of mental health. It's crucial to have safe and encouraging environments in the home, at school, and in the community at large.

Many factors affect mental health. The more risk factors adolescents are exposed to, the greater the potential effect on their mental health. Some factors that can contribute to stress during the adolescence stage include exposure to adversity, pressure to fit into peers, and exploration of identity. Social media influence and gender norms can exacerbate the disparity between an adolescent's lived reality and their perceptions or aspirations for the future. Other important determinants include the quality of their home life and relationships with peer groups. Violence (especially bullying and sexual violence), harsh parenting and severe and socioeconomic problems are recognized as risks to mental health.

Some adolescents are at greater risk of mental health disorders due to their way of living, stigma, discrimination or exclusion, or lack of access to quality support and services. These include adolescents living in humanitarian and fragile settings; adolescents with a chronic sickness, autism spectrum disorder, an intellectual disability, or other neurological condition; pregnant adolescents, adolescent parents, or those in forced or early marriages; orphans; and adolescents from minority ethnic or sexual backgrounds or other discriminated groups.

Emotional Disorders

Many adolescents experience emotional issues. The most common problems related to this age group are anxiety disorders, which might include panic attacks or excessive worrying. Older adolescents experience these diseases more frequently than younger ones. Anxiety disorders are thought to affect 3.6% of 10 to 14-year-olds and 4.6% of 15 to 19-year-olds. According to estimates, 2.8% of teenagers aged 15 to 19 and 1.1% of adolescents aged 10 to 14 experience depression. Rapid and unexpected mood triggers are among the symptoms that both depression and anxiety share.

School attendance or academic performance can be greatly impacted by anxiety and depressive disorders. Isolation and loneliness may become the order of the day for such children if social retreat occurs. Depression can easily lead to suicide.

Behavioral Disorders

All children experience behavioral issues at some point in time, and some parents can manage them because they are a very common occurrence. However, assistance should be sought in understanding and resolving the situation so that both the parents and the child in question will be able to manage it when a specific behavior pattern becomes alarming and harmful.

Overactive kids getting into mischief, playing pranks, being occasionally unruly, and other milder behavioral patterns would be the more prevalent, not actually threatening or extremely destructive behavioral problems.

Nevertheless, when these initially less severe patterns take on a more severe and menacing manifestation of negativity, they can no longer be considered usual and should instead be treated as behavioral disorders.

The more frequent warning signs of such negative and frequently destructive behavior would be harming or threatening themselves, pets, or others, managing or destroying property, lying or stealing, performing poorly in school or even skipping classes, using alcohol and other drugs early in life, engaging in sexual activity early in life, having frequent temper outbursts and arguments, and displaying persistent hostility towards authority figures.

All the above displays would certainly indicate a badly behaved child, and the parent would almost always feel at a loss on how to cope in such situations.

The confusion and anger felt by both sides should be dealt with appropriately so that improvement can be made to try and overcome this negative energy and help the child accept the idea of help with the goal of getting back a calmer and better behavior that others can cope with.

Modern studies have been able to demonstrate that unfavorable behavior patterns are occasionally caused by brain disorders rather than just external circumstances.

It is important to consider the possibility that one of the causes of the behavior being observed is a lack of some neurotransmitters or simply chemical imbalances in the brain.

The possibility of suffering behavioral disorders in younger adolescents is more likely than in older teenagers. 3.1% of 10–14-year-olds and 2.4% of 15–

19-year-olds have attention deficit hyperactivity disorder (ADHD), which is characterized by problems paying attention, excessive activity, and behaving without thinking about the consequences (1). 3.6% of 10 to 14-year-olds and 2.4% of 15 to 19-year-olds have conduct disorder, which is characterized by symptoms of destructive or difficult behavior. Adolescents with behavioral problems may struggle academically and may engage in criminal activity.

Birth Defects

Birth defects are usually defined as any predominant abnormalities of structure, function, or body metabolism that may or may not be obvious at the time of birth.

The relevant support teams will be able to help the parents, in the case of the more obvious abnormalities, either learn how to live with the birth defect or explore other alternatives available to correct the issue as soon as it is legal.

The main focus of structural or metabolic problems would be on particular body parts that are either missing or malformed in some way and may result from a chemistry-related issue that prevented the development of a complete and ideal kid in the womb.

Eating Disorders
Eating disorders, such as anorexia nervosa and bulimia nervosa, commonly appear during adolescence and early adulthood. An eating disorder is described by unusual eating habits and obsession with food, which are commonly accompanied by worries about one's appearance and weight. Anorexia nervosa has a greater death rate than any other mental condition, and it can result in early death, often through medical complications or suicide.

Psychosis
Psychotic symptoms-containing conditions typically first appear in early adulthood. Hallucinations and delusions are examples of signs of psychosis. These experiences can ruin an adolescent's capability to participate in daily activities and education and often lead to stigmatization or human rights violations.

Suicide and Self-Harm
For older teens, suicide is the fourth-leading cause of mortality (15-19 years). There are different types of risk factors for suicide, such as excess alcohol intake,

being molested as a child, being branded for asking for help, struggling to get care, and having access to means of suicide.

Risk-Taking Behaviors

The adolescence stage is when many health-risky activities like substance use and immoral sexual experimentation begin. Risk-taking behaviors can have a negative impact on an adolescent's mental and physical health and can be an unhelpful coping mechanism for emotional troubles.

Males were particularly at risk, with a 13.6% global prevalence of heavy episodic drinking among adolescents aged 15 to 19 in 2020.

Other issues include cannabis and cigarette use. Many smokers started their habit before attaining the age of 18 years old. Cannabis is the most commonly used drug among adolescents, with 4.7% of those aged 15 to 16 reporting using it.

Violence is a risk-taking behavior that can raise the possibility of poor educational performance, injury, criminal activity, or even death. Interpersonal violence was one of the main causes of death among older adolescent boys.

CHAPTER FOUR

Early Detection and Treatment

Taking care of the needs of young people with mental health concerns is essential. Avoiding institutionalization and over-medication, giving non-pharmacological methods top priority, and upholding children's rights in accordance with the United Nations Convention on the Rights of the Child and other human rights agreements are all necessary for promoting adolescents' mental health.

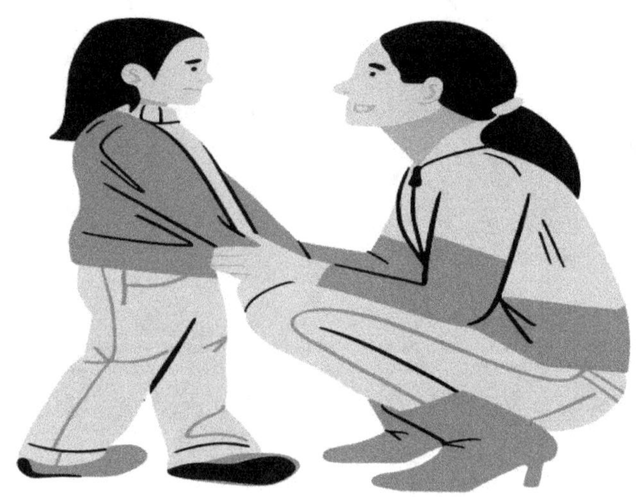

Can Childhood Mental Disorders Be Treated?

Mental disorders in children can be managed and treated. Based on the greatest and most recent medical research, there are many therapy alternatives available. Those involved in the child's care, including teachers, coaches, therapists, and other family members, should work in partnership closely with parents and doctors. By exploiting all the available resources at their disposal, parents, medical professionals, and educators can help the child succeed. Children with mental issues can have better lives with an early diagnosis and the required services for them and their family.

The Impacts of mental disorders in children
Mental disorders in children can be managed and treated. Based on the greatest and most recent medical research, there are numerous therapy alternatives. Everyone involved in the child's care, including teachers, coaches, therapists, and other family members, should work closely with parents and doctors. By utilizing all the legal available resources, parents, medical experts, and educators can help the child succeed. Children's lives can be affected by early diagnosis and appropriate services for kids and their families. The state of one's mind affects their

physical well-being. Mental disorders are long-lasting and frequently persistent health issues that might last the entirety of a person's life. Children with mental disorders may experience difficulties at home, in school, and in other areas without prompt diagnosis and treatment.

What you can do?
- ❖ **Parents:** The best person to judge your child is you. If you are worried about how your child is acting at home, school, or with friends, speak to a healthcare provider.

- ❖ **Youth:** Just as crucial as maintaining good physical health is maintaining good mental health. Never be afraid to speak out to a trusted friend or an adult if you are feeling upset, anxious, or angry.

- ❖ **Healthcare professionals:** Early diagnosis and effective treatment based on current recommendations are crucial. There are resources available to assist in the diagnosis and treatment of mental disorder in children.

* **Teachers/school administrators:** It's critical to make an early diagnosis so that kids can obtain the support they require. If you are worried about a student's mental health at your school, work with the family and medical specialists.

Signs a child might be struggling

Many children and teenagers will eventually struggle with emotional or behavioral issues. While some will pass with time, others will require professional assistance.

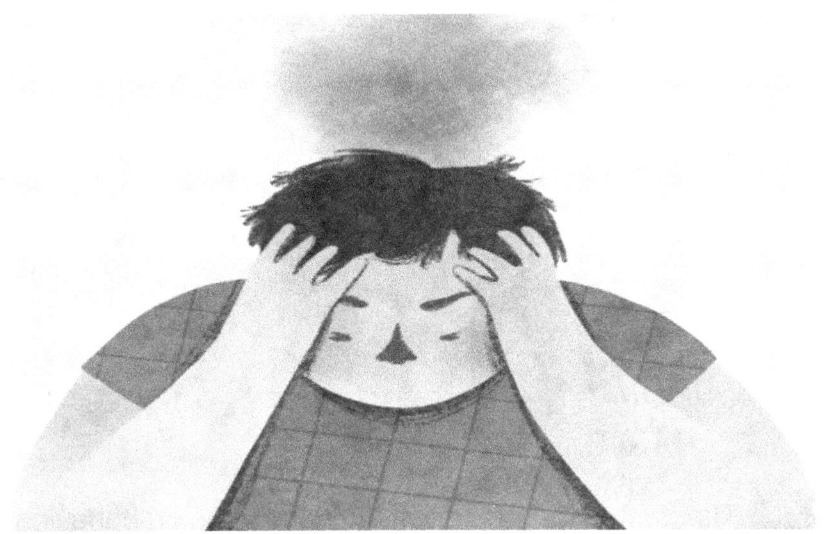

It might be difficult to know if there is something upsetting your child, but there are ways to spot when something's wrong. Watch out for:

> Significant changes in behavior
> Ongoing difficulty sleeping
> Withdrawing from social situations
> Not wanting to do things they usually like
> Self-harm or neglecting themselves

When to seek help

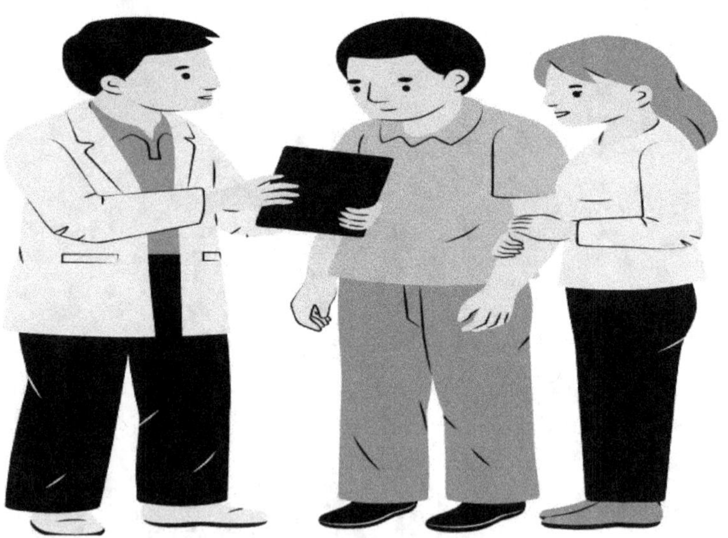

The first people to identify emotional or behavioral issues in a child are frequently their parents and other family members. You can decide to get your child's help after comparing your observations with those of teachers and other caregivers. See your child's physician or a mental health professional if you believe there may be an issue or if you have any questions.

Warning Signs

The following signs may indicate the need for professional assistance or evaluation:

Decline in school performance

Poor grades despite strong efforts

Regular worry or anxiety

Repeated refusal to go to school or take part in normal children's activities

Hyperactivity or fidgeting

Persistent nightmares

Persistent disobedience or aggression

Frequent temper tantrums

Depression, sadness or irritability

Where to Seek Help

Information and referrals regarding the types of services that are available for children may be obtained from:

Mental health organizations, hotlines and libraries

Other professionals such as the school counselor or child's pediatrician

Other families in the community

Family network organizations

Community-based psychiatric care

Crisis outreach teams

Education or special education services

Family resource centers and support groups

Health services

Protection and advocacy groups and organizations

Self-help and support groups

What Does Psychology Have To Offer?

The development of more effective programs for children and families in terms of promotion, prevention, and treatment has been aided by psychological research. These programs include initiatives that target expectant mothers, kids in educational settings, and kids growing up, as well as initiatives that operate on the following levels:

- ❖ **Individual** (e.g., therapy or counseling for those with mental health disorders)
- ❖ **Peer** (e.g., peer-assisted learning programs aimed at improving reading, math, and science)
- ❖ **Family** (e.g., parent education on the needs of children at each stage of development)
- ❖ **School** (e.g., strategies for teachers supporting social and emotional development)
- ❖ **Community** (e.g., violence prevention programs administered through community/recreational centers or churches)
- ❖ **Systemic** (e.g., coordination of services in the health, juvenile justice, education, and child protection systems)

❖   Psychologists working with children are also trained to consider developmental pathways for:

- ✓ *Identity*
- ✓ *Emotions*
- ✓ *Social engagement*
- ✓ *Cognition*

Physical and mental development Children's behavior is also greatly influenced by culture, ethnicity, and language, which has an impact on how mental health is promoted and how mental health illnesses are prevented and treated.

Psychologists have created instruments to evaluate for behavioral or emotional issues, provide therapy when necessary, and continuously track the effectiveness of treatment. They have also developed assessments to assess the risk and protective variables for children's mental health.

Additionally, psychologists have created programs that successfully involve families, schools, and communities—the crucial social supports that help ensure children's long-term wellbeing. For example, one effective family-centered program that aims to reduce pre-teen alcohol use involves parents and other caregivers by teaching them how to be good parents, including how to set limits, communicate clearly about substance abuse, and be disciplined. Children are also taught how to resist alcohol and how to develop negative attitudes toward it.

How does one find a psychologist for children?

Psychologists working with children can be found in many settings:

- ✓ In schools
- ✓ In community health centers
- ✓ In hospitals working in partnership with pediatricians and psychiatrists
- ✓ In research centers
- ✓ In private practice

Promotion and prevention of mental health

Interventions for mental health promotion and prevention seek to improve an individual's capacity for emotion regulation, strengthen substitutes to risk-taking behaviors, foster flexibility for dealing with trouble and difficult situations, and advance fostering of social environments and social networks.

These programs require a multi-level strategy with various delivery channels, such as digital media, health or social care facilities, schools, or the community, as well as various approaches to reach young people, especially the most vulnerable ones.

Various evidence has suggested that mental health and its determinants can be improved in association with planned or unplanned changes in the social and physical environment.

Health promotion has been defined as action and advocacy to address the full range of potentially modifiable determinants of health (WHO 1998). Health promotion and prevention are essentially interconnected and overlapping activities. Because mental health promotion is concerned with the determinants of health while mental health prevention focuses on the causes of disease, promotion is often used as an umbrella concept covering also the more specific activities of prevention.

DIGITAL MENTAL HEALTH INTERVENTION FOR CHILDREN AND PARENTS

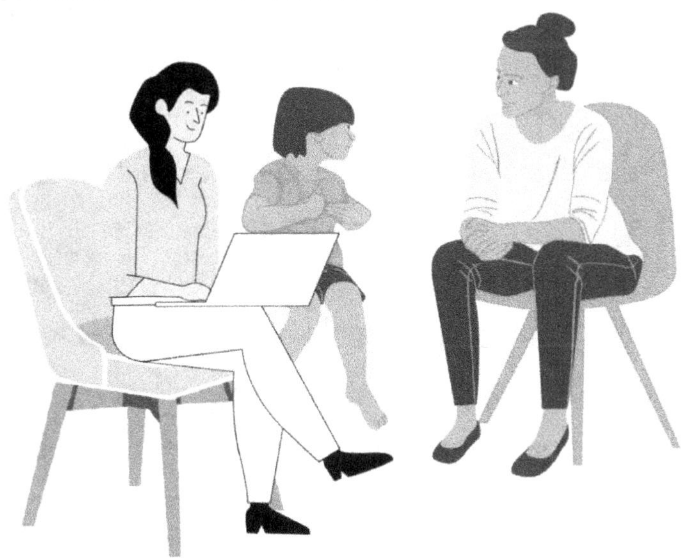

The number of children with mental health difficulties is increasing; as a result, over 850,000 youngsters in the UK are thought to have clinically significant problems, with just a quarter displaying signs of mental illness. Family members frequently find it difficult to deal with children who have mental health issues. As a result, people looking for professional mental health care are increasingly turning to digital mental health solutions. According to some research, parents who are divorced or working away from home find it difficult to keep in touch with their children. This gap in communication between parents and their children might worsen the children's mental health problems and hinder early diagnosis. There are few people looking for professional services in recent years, it can be seen that there is an increase in health-related applications delivered through mobile and desktop devices to support the management of chronic health conditions. Thus, digital mental health interventions are getting widespread for low-help-seeking people to help access professional mental health services. Undoubtedly, technological advances in treatment are not limited to web-based programs, yet socially assisted robotics (SAR), which is among the new and developing technology-based treatment options, has developed.

Working parents have a unique set of challenges as they attempt to balance work and family duties. About 75% of parents struggle to balance work and family life. There are numerous therapies available to help parents overcome this.

Digital mental health interventions (DMHI) have the potential to benefit everyone, especially people with intellectual disabilities, as a complement to therapy, but not as a replacement for face-to-face services, as the perceived value of in-person support for a therapist came through the responses.

The mobile health (MHealth) application, Zingo is one of those numerous applications designed to promote therapy activities for children aged between 6 and 12 years living with neurodevelopmental disabilities. It is suitable for children with a broad range of neurodevelopmental disabilities, including cerebral palsy and autism spectrum disorder, although some children living with more severe disabilities may require additional assistance when using the app.

AI and Emotion Detection

Artificial intelligence (AI) is the replication of human insights in robots that have been made to think and act like humans. Emotional AI refers to technologies that detect, learn about, and associate with human emotional life using effective computing and artificial intelligence methodologies. According to current data, the high frequency of mental illness and, as a result, the need for efficient mental health care, along with later advances in AI, have resulted in an increase in the study of how the machine learning (ML) sector might aid in diagnostics, determination, and treatment.

CHAPTER FIVE

What Every Child Needs for Good Mental Health

Parents can easily recognize a child's bodily needs, which include a nutritious meal, suitable clothing during cold weather, and a reasonable bedtime. Nonetheless, the child's cognitive and emotional needs might not be as obvious. Children with healthy mental growth are better equipped to think critically, develop their social skills, and learn new skills. Kids must also surround themselves with encouraging individuals and great companions if they are to grow in self-assurance, strong self-esteem, and a healthy emotional outlook on life.

A child's physical and mental health are both important.

Basics for a child's good physical health:

- Nutritious food
- Adequate shelter and sleep
- Exercise
- Immunizations
- Healthy living environment
- Unconditional love from family

- Self-confidence and high self-esteem

- The opportunity to play with other children

- Encouraging teachers and supportive caretakers

- Safe and secure surroundings

- Appropriate guidance and discipline

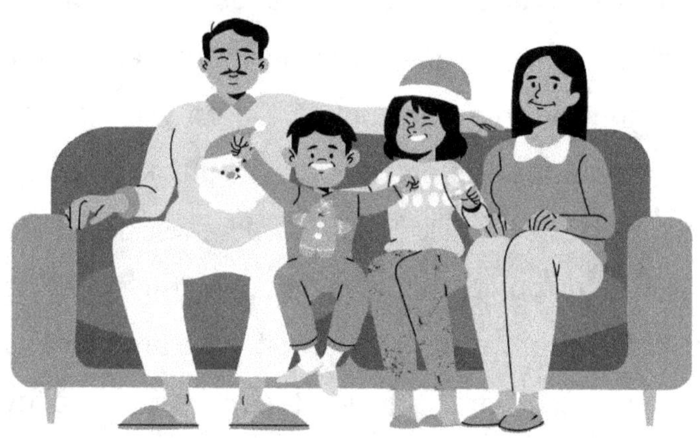

Give children unconditional love.

The three priorities of every family should be love, security, and acceptance. Children must know that your affection for them is unconditional and unconnected to their achievements.

Failures and/or mistakes must be anticipated and acknowledged. In a home that is filled with unending love and affection, confidence grows.

Encourage children's confidence and self-esteem.

Praise Them: Children gain a desire to explore and learn about their environment when their first steps or aptitude for learning a new game is encouraged. Let kids to play and explore in a protected place where they won't get hurt. Ensure them by grinning and interacting with them more frequently. Participate actively in their activities. Their sense of self-worth and confidence are enhanced by your attention.

Set Realistic Goals - Children need realistic goals that match their goals with their abilities. With your assistance, older children can select activities that test their abilities and increase their self-confidence.

Be Honest – always tell your children the truth and don't hide your mistakes from them. They need to understand that nobody is perfect, errors are something we all make. Acknowledging that grownups make mistakes may be incredibly reassuring.

Avoid Sarcastic Statements - Ask the child how they feel about the scenario if they miss a game or fail an exam. Youngsters could become dejected and want encouragement. When they are ready, speak up and reassure them later.

Encourage children: children should put up their best effort while also taking pleasure in the process. Children learn about teamwork, self-esteem, and new skills as they partake in new activities.

Encourage Children to Play: Children view play as pure amusement. Yet, just like food and proper care, playtime is essential for their development. Kids learn creativity, problem-solving techniques, and self-control through play. Running around and shouting while engaging in vigorous play is not only entertaining for kids, but it also promotes their physical and mental wellbeing.

Children Need Playmates: Children should occasionally spend time with their peers. Children establish their feeling of belonging, identify their talents and flaws, and learn how to get along with others through playing with other kids. Think about asking your neighbors, local community centers, schools, or your park and recreation agency for recommendations on a good kids' program.

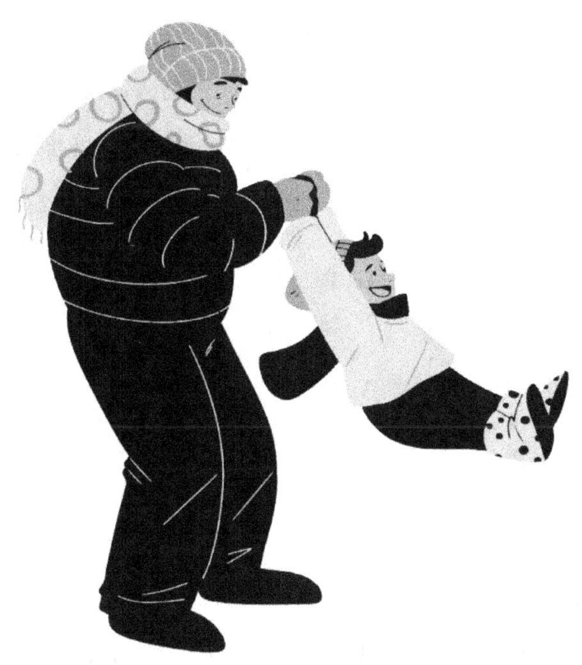

Playing Monopoly or drawing together with children is a great way to exchange ideas and enjoy some quality time.

Play for Pleasure: Being involved and having fun is more important than winning. Did you having fun? is one of the most best questions to ask kids when having fun. not "Did you succeed?"

In our goal-oriented culture, we often celebrate success and victory. Children who are learning and experimenting with new things may find this approach disheartening and irritating. **TV use should be**

monitored: Try to avoid frequently using TV to "baby-sit." Choose children's television programs carefully. Some shows can be enlightening and as well as entertaining.

School should be entertaining: For kids, starting school is an important occasion that calls for celebration. Giving kids a taste of school life by having them play in school can be impactful positively in them.

A pre-school, Head Start, or other comparable community program that offers the chance to interact with other children and develop new friends is something you should try to enroll them in. Also, children can learn the fundamentals of academics as well as decision-making and problem-solving skills.

Provide appropriate guidance and instructive discipline

Children should be given the opportunity to experiment, learn new things, and become self-governing. Children also need to understand that they are responsible for their actions and that some behaviors are intolerable.

Children must learn the norms of the family as members of one. Provide fair and consistent direction and discipline. These social skills and moral principles will follow them to school and eventually the workplace.

Suggestions on Guidance and Discipline

* ***Be firm***, yet be reasonable and polite in your demands. Your love and encouragement are essential to a child's development.

* ***Set a good example,*** If you don't engage in this conduct yourself, you cannot expect a youngster to do so.

* **Criticize the behavior, not the child.** Instead of saying "You are a horrible kid or girl," it is preferable to say "That was a bad thing you did."

* **Avoid nagging, threats and bribery.** Nagging is something that kids will learn to ignore, and bribery and threats rarely work.

* Explain to kids "why" you are punishing them and any possible negative effects of their behavior.

* **Talk about your feelings.** We all experience occasional rage. It's crucial to discuss what

happened and your anger if you do "blow your top." If you were wrong, apologize!

❖ **Provide a safe and secure home.**

It's acceptable for kids to experience fear occasionally. Everybody experiences some form of fear throughout their lives. Anxiety and fear are experiences that we don't fully comprehend.

Finding out what is frightening your kids is the first step if they have persistent anxieties that are influencing their behavior. Be kind, patient, and comforting; avoid being judgmental. Keep in mind that a child's terror could be quite genuine to them.

CHAPTER SIX

Cultural diversity and mental health needs

What is Cultural Diversity?

The cultural diversity meaning is an ideological belief upheld in societies that recognize, appreciate, and respect the cultural behaviors and presence of other people or people from diversified groups. People from a variety of various ethnic backgrounds make up societies. The unique values, behaviors, and social norms of each ethnic group place restrictions on it. Therefore, a culturally diverse society allows and empowers different contributions that different people make from various ethnic backgrounds.

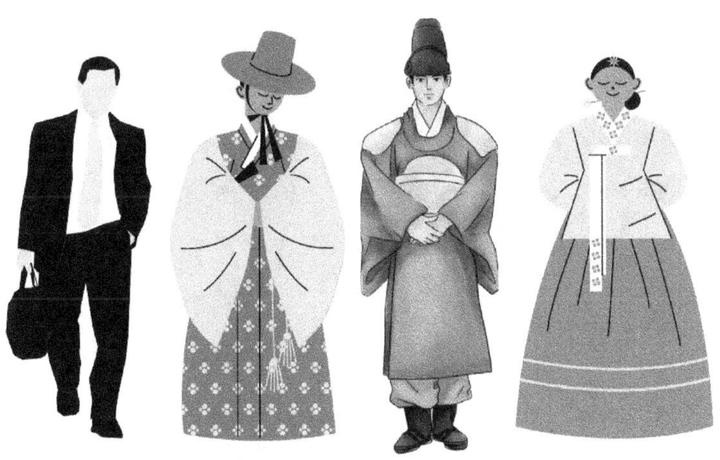

Essentially, cultural diversity is the act of inclusiveness; that is, acknowledging people from different cultural backgrounds and creating an enabling environment that recognizes and values the social behaviors of others. Understanding diversity stands out as a critical aspect of promoting cultural diversity. In this regard, diversity is attributed to various factors such as religion, ethnicity, and race, among others.

In today's culture, cultural diversity encourages peaceful cohabitation between various groups of people. Outstanding traits contribute to the understanding of cultural variety.

The main features of cultural diversity

Existence of Multiple Cultures
The population of the world is made up of people from many civilizations. As a result, in a society that is culturally diverse, there are people from different cultures present, and each of those cultures is the result of individual evolution. The historical evolution of the culture, the individuals engaged, their social interactions, and the population's blending or migration into their contemporary civilization are all

examples of individual growth. Nonetheless, despite coming from various cultural origins, they coexist peacefully and respect one another's differences in culture.

Each Culture has its Distinctive Features

Every culture has distinctive elements that set it apart from others. History, language, the arts, and religion are frequently used characteristics to distinguish one culture from another. Even though each culture has its distinctive basic traits, people continue to live according to their own traditions while also recognizing those of other cultures. Recognizing other people's cultural customs lessens cultural tensions and promotes peaceful coexistence.

It Tries to Preserve

Social customs, religion, cultural traditions, and language all make up a person's culture. Diversity in culture enhances the likelihood that some people will embrace other lifestyles. Yet, when a society recognizes cultural variety, the minority group's culture is urged to protect itself, averting cultural extinction. Recognizing the minority culture's presence and social customs encourages them to carry on practicing their culture, lowering the likelihood of its extinction.

Elements that show the diversity of culture
Every culture has its own unique way of living in a given multicultural setting. Therefore, fundamental elements serve as a pillar of distinguishing the abundant diversity of cultures in modern societies. Some of these elements include:

- ❖ **Languages**
  Language is the means of communicating with another individual. Even if there could be a language barrier, especially when conversing or corresponding with someone from a different cultural background, it is crucial to employ the right strategies to aid advance understanding between the two. For instance, sign language lowers language barriers or employs a language that both parties can easily grasp.

- ❖ **Customs**
  Every culture, or a person within a certain culture, exhibits a distinct behavioral pattern during social interactions. Moreover, beliefs held by members of a particular culture are included in customs.

Hence, respecting other people's traditions is crucial.

❖ Social values

Social values describe the appropriate behavior in a certain social situation. Social values include how people treat others, especially the elderly, how they address those in authority, how kind they are, and how truthful they are. Respect for cultural diversity is aided by social principles.

❖ Social organization

The basic unit of any culture is the family. Therefore, in every culture, a family has its definite obligations. In addition, the social organization also entails dietary needs, product or service preferences, and mutual obligations within the society. Social organization is essential since it helps to bring harmony among its people. It also helps to promote interaction between people from different cultures.

❖ Gender interaction

In cultural settings, gender interaction refers to respect accord to a specific gender or how individuals from different genders interact.

However, in the modern world, gender interaction may be a minor element since most cultures promote fair or equal treatment between the two genders. Nevertheless, some cultures still uphold their traditions. Thus, both men are treated otherwise regarding respect, governance, and mode of interaction.

Benefits of Cultural Diversity

In the modern world, there are various benefits associated with cultural diversity. The main key benefits of cultural diversity include:

Cultural diversity helps promote peaceful coexistence among people from different cultures and ethnicity in their workplace, institutions, and social settings.

Cultural diversity helps people to acknowledge that the world is made up of different types of people from different cultural settings

Cultural diversity helps promote respect for other cultures and learn how they function and live.

There is beauty in promoting cultural diversity in society since people learn new skills from others and encourage innovation through dialogue and consultations.

Cultural diversity is beneficial to people living in the society since it promotes cross-cultural relationship, increases comfort, reduces cultural stereotypes, and impacts positive attitudes toward people living in a given society.

Challenges of Cultural Diversity
Even though cultural diversity is very much practiced in modern society, there are various challenges that are accompanying it. Some of the challenges include:

Language and communication

In some cases, language can be a major barrier for families who change environment. Difficulties in communicating with English can challenging for families and undermine people's confidence. This may make it difficult for job seekers and makes learning at school more difficult, and contribute to social isolation. Language skills can make communication with schools and other services more difficult for parents and careers. Communication issues arise in other ways as well. If the experiences, customs and beliefs of children and families from different cultural backgrounds are not recognized or valued, it creates a huge gap in communication. For example, while greeting prostrating to someone else may be considered a sign of respect in some cultures; however, in some other cultures respect is shown by lowering eyes or looking away. If these variances are not understood by both people, it can lead to miscommunication and misunderstanding on both sides. It is very crucial for families to have access to support in languages they are comfortable with and are able to develop their communication skills if they so desire.

Migration and resettlement

Some families migrate from one country, region or place and settle in another for many reasons. Some families may migrate because they fear they will be harmed and victimized against; they might willingly leave their country of origin to live in another country; or they might leave a country and ask to be recognized as a refugee to be protected. Resettling in a new country or community can be challenging in some cases. Families need to find housing, schools, employment, social connections and services. Lack of knowledge about how things work in the new environment and communication difficulties can make the challenge of resettlement more stressful.

Effects of trauma

When migration is prompted by certain stressful experiences, as is the case for refugees, there can be further challenges for resettlement and wellbeing. Traumatic experiences may have happened through being exposed to violence, torture or war. Children and families may have lived under danger and in fear; they may have witnessed the loss of relatives or friends, or experienced hardship and danger due to change of environment. Some have received cruel treatment in immigration detention on their arrival. These kinds of highly stressful circumstances can have a long-time effect on people after the events have passed. Some of the common reactions that may occur in children who have been through traumatic events include an increase in fear and anxiety, which may lead to clingy behavior, re-experiencing the shock when feeling threatened, or difficulty in believing and relating with others. Such difficulties may lead to children experiencing difficulties trusting others, making it more difficult for them to form relationships with adults or with their peers. For some children who have been traumatized, feelings of pain and anger can sometimes be seen in their behavior, for instance, some children may tantrum or show high levels of emotional reactivity (eg become upset very easily). Difficulties related with past trauma and resettlement can upset the learning and school performance of children who have been traumatized.

Discrimination and racism

Some people use hurtful words and act poorly against others to cope with their anxieties and lack of knowledge about differences. This is known as discrimination. Discrimination has a harmful influence on both people and whole societies. Several persons from various backgrounds may suffer difficulties as a result of prejudice. This may be especially problematic for minority groups, such as individuals who appear different from the majority of a community. Direct discrimination (such as name-calling and bullying) and indirect discrimination (such as ignoring or excluding others from significant occasions) may both leave people feeling alone and helpless. This can have a detrimental effect on one's mental health and well-being. Racism makes children feel different and vulnerable by denigrating their culture and making them feel unwelcome. Racism and prejudice may make life more difficult for families, causing unnecessary stress and socioeconomic disadvantage. Respect for diversity and inclusion also promotes respectful interactions and minimizes the possibility of prejudice and isolation.

Parenting in different cultures

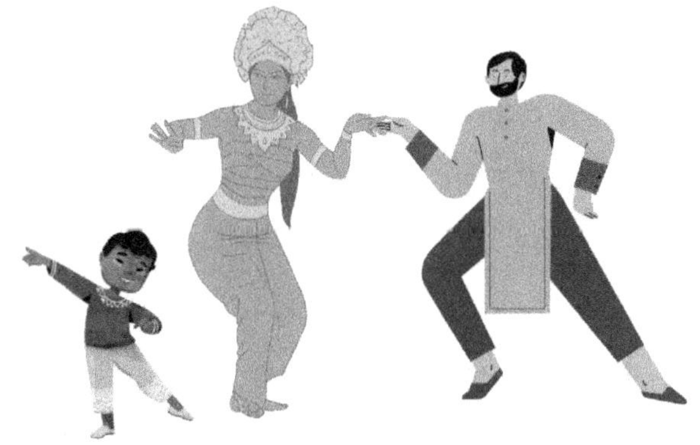

Ethnic disparities in parenting techniques can cause confusion and stress for families. Common disparities in parenting techniques may be attributed to how children are offered love, attitudes toward physical punishment, and how much emphasis is placed on family responsibilities and developing children's independence. Some cultural traditions may have highly severe norms of behavior based on age and/or gender.

The role of schools

Schools are extremely important in the lives of kids and their families. Schools must understand the specific situations of kids and their families from varied backgrounds in order to address their learning, social, and wellness requirements. They may include migration, refugee, and resettlement experiences, as well as various cultural values and communication and learning methods. Schools may play an important role in assisting and engaging kids and families from a variety of backgrounds. Teachers also have a significant obligation to foster mutual tolerance and understanding, as well as to properly handle discriminatory issues in the school context. By aggressively supporting the needs and interests of students and families from culturally diverse backgrounds, as well as developing trusting and understanding relationships with parents and caregivers. A positive feeling of belonging allows children to cope with cultural variety more easily and confidently, and it boosts their motivation and involvement at school. School personnel may help students by respecting and understanding their unique backgrounds and cultural identities (including specific behavioral and communication requirements). Children and their families feel more at ease and valued at school under these settings.

Developing relationships

To enhance children's well-being, developing cross-cultural interactions necessitates strong communication and flexibility. It is also crucial to remember that various cultures may have quite diverse understandings of mental health and a variety of ways of communicating difficulties. Children's emotional or behavioral difficulties, for example, should be recognized in the context of their cultural environment and handled with families in a helpful and nonjudgmental manner. Good interactions between families and school personnel demonstrate tolerance for diversity while also improving children's mental health and well-being.

Overcoming Diversity Challenges

Diversity and inclusion are indisputable components of long-term company success, and the organization should embrace this trend.

If the aforementioned issues are not addressed effectively, the process may become unpleasant. These are some suggestions for making your workplace more equal and inclusive.

Each employee's different background and experiences should be valued by the firm. To counteract the monotony of "sameness," varied points of view generate fresh perspectives. Companies should endeavor to understand diversity ideals and continually expand employee awareness of the problem.

Managers and team leaders must provide equal and transparent opportunities for their team members to communicate and submit suggestions for development. Each employee must feel heard and valued for who they are and what they are capable of. These unusual events are critical for teams to develop a climate receptive to invention.

Every culture should be acknowledged and appreciated in the same way. Express clearly that no one can fully know another person's background, but that everyone is willing to learn. As a result, rather than conforming to the majority, everyone should be given the opportunity to offer their ideas. You may increase communication by considering each employee as an individual rather than as a group.

Take a stance

Being neutral is no longer a reasonable decision since it may bring more harm than benefit. Workers would believe that the company is not treating them fairly and is instead acting ambiguously.

Managers must be kept up to date on current developments in order to act fast. Nowadays, a variety of cultural issues, such as Black Lives Matter and gender inequality, are causing worry.

Make better use of diversity

Two-thirds of employees said that diversity was essential to them when evaluating firms and employment offers, according to numerous surveys. In other words, businesses would stand out more in the crowded job market if they could demonstrate that they are fostering a diverse and inclusive culture.

Every person in a varied firm have unique characteristics and abilities that others might benefit from. Every day, when people are exposed to different cultures, methods of doing things, and points of view, they should be given the opportunity to grow and learn.

What matters more is how firms can combine cooperation initiatives and link staff development plans with the company's goal to ensure sustainability. As a result, the next critical step is to develop an action plan to put all of the aforementioned concepts into action.

Why Does Cultural Diversity Matter When Considering, Identifying And Addressing Mental Health Needs In Our Community?

Because of the complicated link between cultural diversity and the needs of the community in terms of mental health, it is vital to include cultural diversity when defining and satisfying these requirements. Culture may have a negative impact on mental health since it directly influences how you perceive particular ideas or actions. It can have an influence on a variety of things, including whether or not you seek treatment for mental health difficulties. Because of the complicated link between cultural diversity and the needs of the community in terms of mental health, it is vital to include cultural diversity when defining and satisfying these requirements. Because culture has a direct impact on mental health, it can have a variety of negative implications. It can affect a variety of things, including whether you decide to seek treatment for mental health problems or not, as well as other things.

It's important that we understand the role culture plays in mental health care so we can support our loved ones and encourage treatment when it's needed most.

Ways Culture Can Impact Mental Health:

Cultural Stigma

Every culture has a unique perspective on and attitude toward mental health. In some cultures, asking for help when you need it is viewed as "weakness," and people may feel pressured to keep their mental health problems hidden. These incorrect assumptions about mental health might make it difficult for people to obtain assistance and freely talk about their concerns.

Understanding Symptoms

A person's culture also has an impact on how they view and feel about their symptoms. In some countries, admitting you have symptoms of a mental health issue might be embarrassing. Furthermore, how people accept their symptoms is influenced by culture. Some people may prefer to concentrate primarily on certain symptoms. For example, someone from a certain culture can elect to choose to only notice and talk about physical issues rather than emotional ones since that is what their society encourages.

Community Support

A person's culture also has an influence on how they see and feel about their symptoms. Admitting you have signs of a mental health problem can be embarrassing in some cultures. Additionally, how people accept their symptoms is impacted by culture. Some individuals may choose to focus on specific symptoms solely. A person from one culture, for instance, might opt to solely recognize and converse with individuals from that culture. The level of support a person receives during a mental health crisis may vary depending on cultural factors. Depending on cultural factors, people may be forced to seek out mental health treatments and support on their own for physical symptoms rather than emotional ones when thcy express concerns about their mental health.

Resources

Culture can have an influence on how to use the resources for mental health. The urge to acquire mental health treatment from someone with a comparable experience to you is regular and legitimate. As supporters of mental health, we respect the unique perspectives that diverse cultures may provide. We are aware that views on mental health and mental health concerns might vary between cultures. By being aware of how culture influences mental health

MENTAL HEALTH AND HUMAN RIGHTS

An environment that respects and defends basic civil, political, economic, social, and cultural rights is vital to the promotion of mental health. It is exceedingly challenging to maintain a high level of mental health without the safety and freedom that these rights afford.

A human rights framework offers a useful tool for identifying and addressing the underlying determinants of mental health. A collection of globally recognized values and concepts that can direct nations in the development, implementation, monitoring, and assessment of mental health policies, regulations, and initiatives can be found in the components of the United Nations (UN) human rights framework. They create responsibility for mental health and provide a helpful benchmark by which to measure government performance in the promotion of mental health since they are legal norms and standards that governments have accepted. By granting them entitlements that result in legal responsibilities on the part of governments, human rights enable individuals and communities to flourish. They can serve to equalize the allocation and exercise of power within society, thereby lessening the helplessness of the poor. The ideals of equality and freedom from discrimination, which are important aspects of the international human rights framework, necessitate that particular attention be paid to vulnerable populations. Furthermore, the right of all people to participate in decision-making processes, which is reflected in the Bill of Rights and other UN instruments, can help ensure that marginalized groups are able to influence health-related matters and strategies that affect them, and that their interests are considered and addressed. The promotion of mental health is not just the responsibility of health ministries. It requires the involvement of a wide range of sectors, actors, and stakeholders. Human rights comprise civil, cultural, economic, political, and social dimensions and so give an intersectional framework to evaluate mental health across the vast spectrum of mental health determinants.

Progress Monitoring For Parents/Guardians

What is progress monitoring?

Progress monitoring is a data collection process that assists in determining whether interventions or treatments are benefiting your child. The Individualized Educational Program (IEP) includes academic, behavioral, or social goals for your child. Graphic graphs and charts are employed to evaluate the efficacy of the therapy.

Why Progress Monitoring is important?

In order to assist your children, achieve their objectives, educators and families may talk about what is working and what isn't by keeping track of their progress.

How can parents/guardians help with progress monitoring?

Advocate

for your child's learning and educational rights by actively communicating with administrators.

Ask questions

Ask questions because you are a valuable part of the process.

Celebrate

Celebrate your child's accomplishments and progress.

Encourage

Encourage your child to do their best.

Share information

Share information or any feedback about your child's progress.

Progress monitor graph and chat for parents/guardians

If your kid has academic, behavioral or social goals within the Individualized Educational Program (IEP), progress monitoring is a data gathering method that helps determine if interventions or therapies are benefitting your child. Graphic graphs and charts are used to measure the success of the treatment.

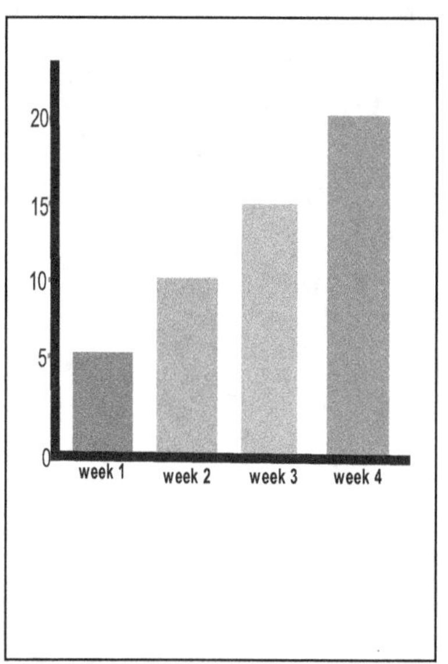
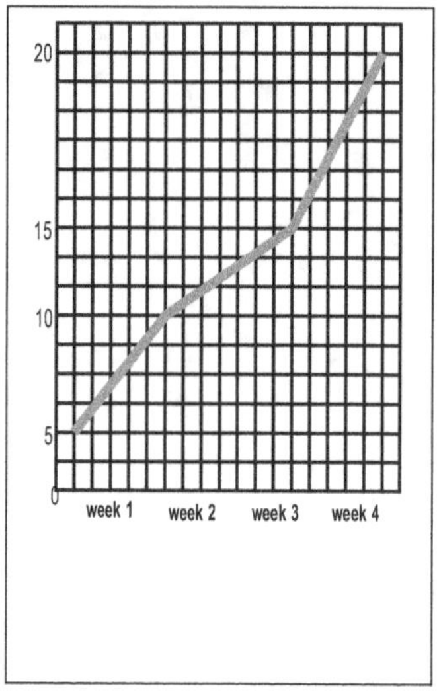

Why is it important?
In order to support child/children meeting their goals, progress monitoring creates accountability and helps

parents/guardians discuss what is working and what is not working.

Journaling

In the space below, reflect on a recent conversation you had with your child about mental health. Print a few copies of this page and try to practice journaling regularly.

Positive aspects of the conversation:

ACTIVITY 1

Positive aspect of the conversation:

Areas to improve on:

Plans for future conversations

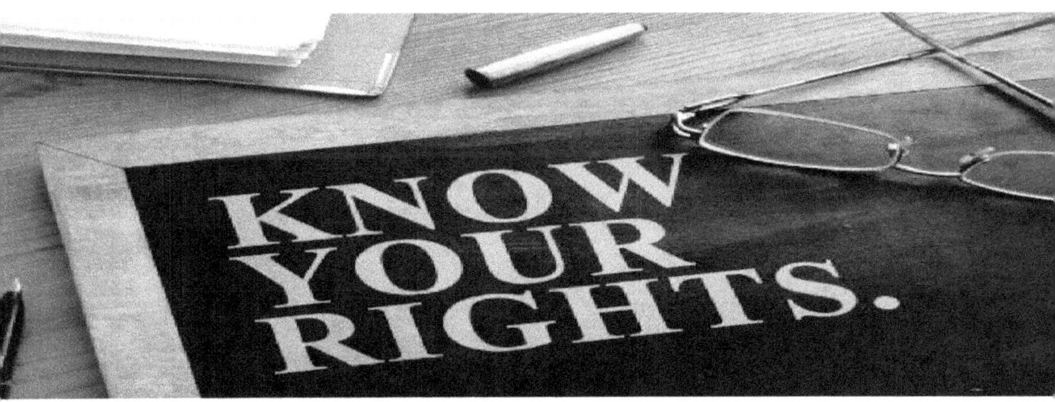

As a parent you have the right to…

Participate
You can assist in the development of your child's individualized education program (IEP) and be educated about alternate   alternatives for your child's special education services

Receive Prior Written Notice
As the school starts your child's educational identification, evaluation, and placement, ask for a written notification in your native tongue.

Access Records
You have the right to access, review, and get copies of your child's educational records Under the Family Educational Rights and Privacy Act (FERPA)

Consent/Refuse Consent

You can accept or decline consent for your child to be assessed and make adjustments in their special education services, and your child's placement

Confidentiality

Parents and guardians are interested in learning about every aspect of their child's existence. As school psychologists and counselors, we have a responsibility to treat our pupils with confidentially. Our confidentiality is violated if your child tells us anything about the following, and you will be informed right away:

- ✓ Threatens to harm themselves
- ✓ Threatens to harm others
- ✓ Threat to a serious crime

ACTIVITY 2

In your own words, tell us what you think is mental health:

____

____

In your own words, tell us what you think is health:

____

In your own words, tell us what you think is cultural diversity:

____

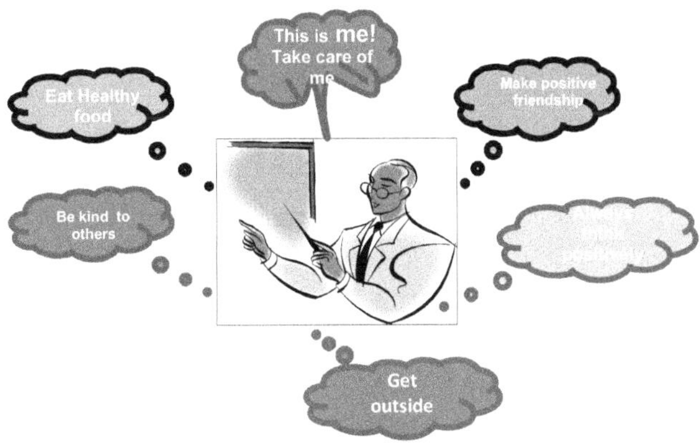

Why take care of your mind?

- ❖ To help live a positive and healthy life

- ❖ To help prevent Mental illness

- ❖ To Help build self-confident

- ❖ To help excel in school

Your health is your wealth! Take proper care of it

ACTIVITY 3

WAYS YOU CAN IMPROVE YOUR MENTAL HEALTH

Some ways we can improve our mental health are:

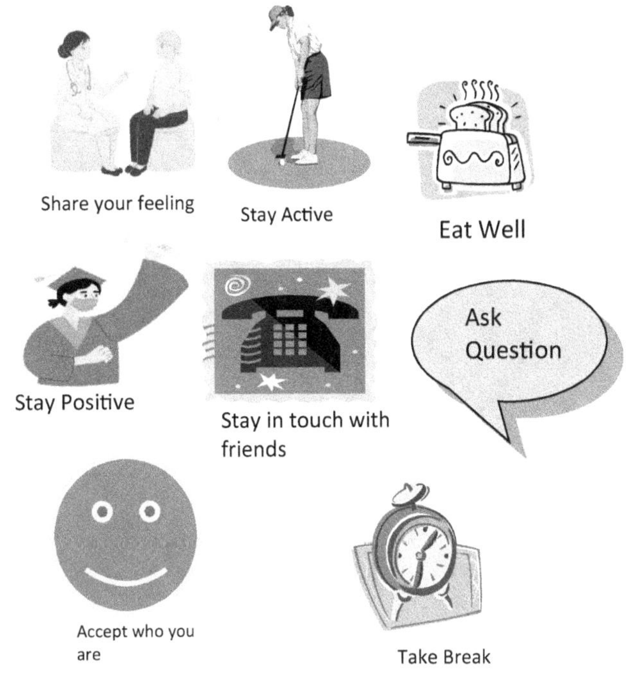

Name some other ways that you take care of your mental health:

1. ___________________________

2. ___________________________

3. ___________________________

4. ___________________________

5. ___________________________

ACTIVITY 4

HOW TO CHECK IN ON YOUR MENTAL HEALTH

One way we can check in on our mental health is by understanding how we feel.

MY FEELINGS

key

Color	I feel this way
	Some times
	Often
	Never

INSTRUCTIONS:

➡ Choose three colors to color in the key

➡ Then look at each feeling in turn

➡ Color in each feeling base on how often you feel this way

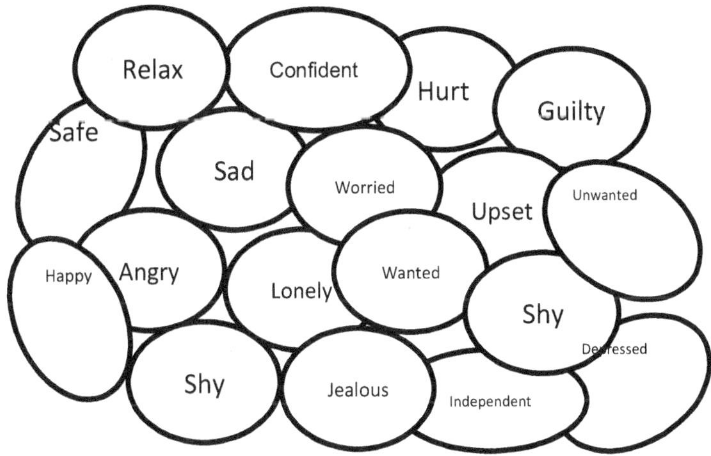

References

https://www.caringforkids.cps.ca/handouts/
mental_health
https://www.mentalhealth.gov/talk/parents-caregivers
https://www.mhanational.org/helping-home-tips-
parents

Kline MV, Huff RM. Health promotion in the context of culture. In Kline MV, and Huff RM editors Health Promotion in Multicultural Populations (2007) (Thousand Oaks: Sage), (pp. 3–22).

UNICEF (2017), How does the time children spend using digital technology impact their mental well-being, social relationships and physical activity? An evidence-focused literature review, https://www.unicef-irc.org/publications/pdf/Children-digital-technology-wellbeing.pdf. [3]

WHO (2003c). Creating an environment for emotional and social wellbeing. Geneva, World Health Organization.

Tones K, Tilford S (2001). Health promotion: effectiveness, efficiency and equity. Cheltenham, Nelson Thornes Ltd.

Mrazek P, Haggerty R, eds (1994). Reducing risks of mental disorder: frontiers for preventive intervention research. Washington, National Academy Press.

Kickbusch I (2003). The contribution of the World Health Organization to a new public health and health promotion. American Journal of Public Health, 93:383–388

WHO (1996). Promoting health through schools. The WHO global school health initiative. Geneva, World Health Organization.

WHO (2002). Prevention and promotion in mental health. Mental health: evidence and research. Geneva, Department of Mental Health and Substance Dependence.

Tomlinson M (2001). A critical look at cultural diversity and infant care. Synergy, Australian Transcultural Mental Health Network, Winter:3–5.

Tang KC, Ehsani J, McQueen D (2003). Evidence based health promotion: recollections, reflections and reconsiderations. Journal of Epidemiology and Community Health, 57:841–843.

www.ingramcontent.com/pod-product-compliance
Lightning Source LLC
Chambersburg PA
CBHW051834250726

48659CB00005B/1834